The Longevity Blueprint

Maximizing Health and Longevity for a Fulfilling Life

by

BARRETT YOUNG

Copyright © by Erik S. Foster 2022. All rights reserved.

Before this document is duplicated or reproduced in any manner, the publisher's consent must be gained. Therefore, the contents within can neither be stored electronically, transferred, nor kept in a database. Neither in Part nor full can the document be copied, scanned, faxed, or retained without approval from the publisher or creator.

TABLE OF CONTENT

Contents

Introduction 5

Understanding the Science of Longevity 5

CHAPTER 1 8

Nutrition for Longevity: The Power of a Healthy Diet 8

CHAPTER 2 11

Exercise for Longevity: Staying Active to Stay Young 11

CHAPTER 3 15

Stress Management for Longevity: Finding Balance in a Busy World.............15

CHAPTER 4 20

Sleep and Longevity: The Importance of Quality Rest 20

CHAPTER 6 29

Relationships and Longevity: Building Strong Connections 29

CHAPTER 6 33

Environmental Factors and Longevity: Living in Harmony with Nature 33

CHAPTER 7 37

Supplements and Longevity: Navigating the World of Anti-Aging 37

Introduction
Understanding the Science of Longevity

The study of longevity focuses on the process of aging as well as the variables that have an effect on the average lifespan of humans. It is a multi-disciplinary area of study that draws from the fields of biology, genetics, medicine, epidemiology, and the social sciences. The study of longevity aims to explain why some people live for a longer period of time than others, as well as to develop ways that can help people live healthier lives for a longer period of time.

The biology of getting older

A complex biological process, aging is characterized by a progressive loss of both physical and mental abilities over the course of one's lifetime. Changes in DNA, oxidative stress, inflammation, and hormonal shifts are thought to be some of the basic mechanisms that lead to aging, however this topic is not fully understood. Genetic factors, lifestyle variables, and environmental factors, including as exposure to chemicals and stress, are also known to have a role in the aging process.

The genes behind a long life

Studies of families with remarkable longevity (those who live to the age of 100 or older) have helped to identify genetic markers that may lead to long life. [Citation needed] The genetics of longevity, on the other hand, are quite complicated, and there is no such thing as a "longevity gene." Instead, it is believed that longevity is the consequence of a large number of different genes interacting with one another as well as with environmental circumstances.

elements related to lifestyle and the environment

The length of one's life can also be significantly impacted by variables such as lifestyle and the surrounding environment. For instance, smoking, having a bad diet, and a lack of physical activity are key risk factors for developing chronic diseases and dying at an early age. On the other side, studies have shown that having a nutritious diet, being physically active on a regular basis, and maintaining a cheerful attitude can all add years to one's life. Living in an environment that is both supportive and socially engaging is another factor that can contribute to healthy aging.

The epidemiology of old age

The study of the occurrence, causes, and factors that contribute to health and disease in communities is referred to as epidemiology. It is utilized to get an understanding of the patterns and causes of diseases and ailments associated with aging, such as cardiovascular disease, cancer, and Alzheimer's disease. Researchers can find techniques for avoiding and controlling these disorders, which can assist to increase lifespans, by investigating the factors that influence these diseases and determining what factors influence them.

The study of how different circumstances can affect a person's lifespan is known as the "science of longevity," and it is an extremely complicated and fast developing topic. Although genetics do play a part in determining longevity, variables related to lifestyle and the environment also play a vital role in the process. By gaining a deeper understanding of the biological, genetic, and environmental components that contribute to aging, we will be better able to devise methods that can assist individuals in living healthier lives for longer periods of time.

CHAPTER 1

Nutrition for Longevity: The Power of a Healthy Diet

Nutrition plays a critical role in promoting longevity and overall health. A healthy diet that includes a balanced mix of essential nutrients and is low in unhealthy foods can help support the body's natural defences against ageing and reduce the risk of chronic diseases. Incorporating a healthy diet into your daily routine can improve mental clarity, boost energy levels, and enhance the overall quality of life.

It is critical to remember that individual nutrient needs may vary based on factors such as age, gender, and health status. Incorporating portion control and balancing caloric intake with physical activity is essential to maintain a healthy weight and to promote longevity.

Incorporating a healthy diet into your lifestyle can also have additional benefits beyond promoting longevity, such as reducing the risk of chronic diseases, improving cardiovascular health, and supporting healthy ageing. Adopting a holistic approach that considers all aspects of your lifestyle, including regular physical activity and stress management techniques, can help to optimize your overall health and well-being.

Remember to seek the advice of a healthcare professional or a registered dietitian to ensure that your diet is tailored to meet your individual needs and goals. With the proper support and resources, you can adopt a healthy and sustainable lifestyle that will support your longevity and overall health for years to come.

Additionally, it's important to keep an open mind and be willing to try new foods and experiment with different dietary styles to find what works best for you. Eating a variety of nutrient-dense foods can help ensure that you are getting all of the essential nutrients your body needs to thrive.

Some examples of nutrient-dense foods that have been linked to promoting longevity include whole grains, fruits and vegetables, lean proteins, and healthy fats such as nuts, seeds, and olive oil. On the other hand, foods high in added sugars, saturated fats, and refined carbohydrates should be limited to support optimal health and longevity.

The power of a healthy diet should not be underestimated when it comes to promoting longevity and overall well-being. By incorporating a balanced mix of essential nutrients and limiting the intake of unhealthy foods, you can support your body's natural defenses against the aging process and live a long and healthy life. With the right support and resources, levels, and the ability to regulate appetite and metabolism. Aim for 7-9 hours of quality sleep each night and adopt good sleep hygiene habits, such as avoiding screens before bed and creating a relaxing sleep environment.

A healthy diet is only one aspect of promoting longevity and overall well-being. A holistic approach that considers all aspects of your lifestyle, including physical activity, stress management, and sleep quality, is necessary to optimize your health and support a long and healthy life. By altering your lifestyle and incorporating healthy routines, you can take control of your health and promote longevity for years to come.

CHAPTER 2

Exercise for Longevity: Staying Active to Stay Young

Exercise plays a critical role in promoting longevity and overall health. Regular physical activity can help to reduce the risk of chronic diseases such as heart disease, stroke, and type 2 diabetes, and also improve mental clarity, boost energy levels, and enhance overall quality of life. By incorporating exercise into your daily routine, you can support your body's natural defenses against the aging process and promote healthy aging.

you can take control of your health and adopt a sustainable and nutritious lifestyle that will serve you for years to come.

The science of longevity and the role that nutrition plays in promoting health and longevity are complex and multifaceted. In addition to a healthy diet, several other lifestyle factors such as physical activity, stress management, and sleep quality can play a significant role in promoting longevity.

Physical activity is essential for good health. can help reduce the risk of chronic diseases such as heart disease, stroke, and type 2 diabetes. Plan to engage in moderate-intensity physical activity for at least 30 minutes. such as brisk walking, every day. Strength training, such as weightlifting, can also be beneficial for promoting healthy aging by building muscle mass and improving bone density.

Stress management is also critical for promoting longevity and overall well-being. Chronic stress can have a negative impact on health, including increasing the risk of heart disease, stroke, and certain types of cancer. practicing disciplines like yoga, meditation, and deep breathing can help manage stress levels and promote relaxation.

Quality sleep is also essential for promoting longevity and overall health. Poor sleep quality can have a negative impact on various aspects of health, including mental clarity, energy

The benefits of exercise for longevity are well-established and numerous. For example, physical activity can help improve cardiovascular health by strengthening the heart and reducing the risk of heart disease. Additionally, it can support blood sugar control and improve insulin sensitivity, which is important for reducing the risk of type 2 diabetes. Exercise has also been shown to reduce the risk of certain types of cancer and improve bone density, helping to reduce the risk of osteoporosis and fractures.

Exercise can also have a positive impact on mental health and well-being. Frequent physical activity has been shown to reduce symptoms of depression, anxiety, and stress, and improve overall mental clarity and cognitive function.

When it comes to exercise for longevity, it's important to find an activity that you enjoy and that you can realistically maintain over time. Some popular options include walking, running, cycling, swimming, and strength training. Get at 30 minutes of moderate physical activity, such as brisk walking, every day, and incorporate strength training into your routine at least twice a week.

It's also important to remember that individual exercise needs may vary based on factors such as age, gender, and health status. Consult with a healthcare professional or fitness professional to determine the best exercise plan for you and to ensure that your routine is tailored to meet your specific needs and goals.

exercise is an essential component of promoting longevity and overall well-being. By incorporating physical activity into your daily routine, you can reduce the risk of chronic diseases, improve mental clarity, and enhance overall quality of life. With the right support and resources, you can adopt a healthy and sustainable exercise routine that will support your longevity and overall health for years to come.

It's also important to note that the type and intensity of exercise that is best for promoting longevity can vary depending on an individual's age and physical health. For example, older adults may benefit from low-impact activities, such as walking or swimming, while younger adults may benefit from higher-intensity activities, such as running or cycling.

In addition to traditional forms of exercise, there are also other forms of physical activity that can be incorporated into your routine to promote longevity. For example, yoga and tai chi are forms of exercise that combine physical activity with mindfulness and stress management, which can have a positive impact on overall well-being.

It's also important to remember that exercise doesn't have to be done all at once. Breaking up your exercise routine into shorter, more manageable segments can be just as effective and can help make exercise a more achievable goal. For example, you could walk for 10 minutes before breakfast, take a lunchtime walk, and then do a yoga session in the evening.

Finally, it's important to remember that while exercise is an essential component of promoting longevity, it's only one piece of the puzzle. A balanced and healthy diet, adequate sleep, and stress management are all critical components of promoting longevity and overall well-being. By adopting a holistic approach to health and wellness, you can support your body's natural defenses against the aging process and promote a long, healthy life.

In conclusion, exercise is a powerful tool for promoting longevity and overall health. By finding an activity that you enjoy and that you can realistically maintain over time, and by adopting a holistic approach to health and wellness, you can support your body's natural defenses against the aging process and promote a long, healthy life for years to come.

CHAPTER 3

Stress Management for Longevity: Finding Balance in a Busy World

A necessary component of modern life is stress, but managing it effectively is essential for promoting longevity and overall health. Chronic stress has been linked to a range of negative health outcomes, including an increased risk of heart disease, depression, and premature death.

There are numerous methods for managing stress that can help to reduce stress and promote relaxation, such as physical exercise, mindfulness meditation, time management, and sleep hygiene. It's important to find the techniques that work best for you and to make them a regular part of your routine.

Physical exercise is one of the most effective stress management techniques, as it has been shown to reduce symptoms of anxiety and depression, improve overall mood, and boost energy levels. Exercise can also help regulate hormones and other physiological processes that are associated with stress, and improve overall physical health.

Mindfulness meditation is another powerful stress management technique, as it involves focusing your attention on the present moment without judgment. This practice has been shown to reduce stress and improve overall mental clarity, making it an effective way to reduce symptoms of anxiety and depression.

Effective time management is critical to stress management, as it can help you prioritize your time and set achievable goals. This can reduce the sense of being overwhelmed and improve work-life balance, leading to reduced stress and improved overall well-being.

Sleep hygiene is also an important component of stress management, as adequate sleep is crucial for both physical and mental well-being. By adopting good sleep habits, such as maintaining a consistent sleep schedule and avoiding screens before bedtime, you can support healthy sleep and reduce stress.

It's also important to remember that individual stress management needs may vary based on factors such as age, gender, and health status. Consult with a healthcare professional or mental health professional to determine the best stress management plan for you and to ensure that your routine is adapted to your particular needs and goals.

Stress management is a critical component of promoting longevity and overall well-being. By adopting effective stress management techniques, such as physical exercise, mindfulness meditation, time management, and sleep hygiene, you can reduce stress, improve overall well-being, and support your body's natural defenses against the aging process. With the right support and resources, you can adopt a healthy and sustainable stress management routine that will support your longevity and overall health for years to come.

In addition to the above-mentioned stress management techniques, there are other strategies that can be effective in reducing stress and promoting longevity. These include:

1. **Social support**: Spending time with family, friends, and other loved ones has been shown to reduce stress and improve overall mental health. Whether through in-person interactions, phone calls, or virtual meetups, connecting with others can be a powerful stress-reliever.

2. **Relaxation techniques**: Deep breathing, yoga, and tai chi are all examples of relaxation techniques that can help reduce stress and promote physical and mental well-being. These practices can help to slow down the body's response to stress, reduce muscle tension, and promote a sense of calm.

3. **Nature exposure**: Spending time in nature has been shown to reduce stress and improve overall mood. Whether through hiking, gardening, or simply spending time in a park, being in nature can help to lower cortisol levels, improve cardiovascular health, and reduce symptoms of anxiety and depression.

4. **Mindful eating**: Eating mindfully, or paying attention to the food you're eating and the sensations it creates in your body, can help to reduce stress and promote overall well-being. Mindful eating can help you to slow down, savor your food, and avoid overeating, which can lead to stress and health problems.

5. **Cognitive-behavioral therapy (CBT)**: CBT is a form of psychotherapy that can be effective in reducing symptoms of anxiety and depression. It involves exploring the thoughts, feelings, and behaviors that contribute to stress and working to change negative patterns.

6. **A healthy lifestyle**: Adopting a healthy lifestyle, including regular physical activity, a balanced diet, and avoiding harmful substances, can help to reduce stress and improve overall health. By taking care of your body and mind, you can reduce the risk of developing stress-related health problems and promote longevity.

It's also important to note that the effects of stress are not just limited to physical and mental health. Stress can also impact social, financial, and professional aspects of life, and it's important to address these areas as well. Consider seeking out the support of a mental health professional or financial advisor if stress is impacting your relationships, finances, or work.

In summary, stress management is a complex and multi-faceted challenge, and a comprehensive approach is needed to address its many impacts. By incorporating a range of stress management techniques, and seeking the support of others when necessary, you can reduce stress, promote longevity, and live a healthy and fulfilling life.

CHAPTER 4

Sleep and Longevity: The Importance of Quality Rest

Sleep is a crucial aspect of overall health and plays an important role in promoting longevity. Lack of sleep, or poor quality sleep, has been linked to a range of health problems, including obesity, heart disease, stroke, and depression. On the other hand, getting adequate, high-quality sleep is essential for maintaining overall health and well-being, and can help to reduce the risk of developing these and other health problems.

Here are some key ways that sleep promotes longevity:

1.**Boosts immune system**: Sleep helps to boost the immune system and reduce the risk of infection. During sleep, the body produces cytokines, which are proteins that help to fight off infections and diseases. Additionally, sleep helps to restore and refresh the immune system, leaving you better prepared to fight off illness and disease.

2.**Regulates hormones**: Sleep is essential for regulating hormones that impact metabolism, appetite, and mood. For example, lack of sleep can disrupt the balance of hormones such as cortisol, which regulates stress, and leptin, which regulates appetite. By ensuring that these hormones are properly regulated, sleep can help to maintain overall health and well-being.

3.**Improves brain function**: Sleep is critical for maintaining brain function, including memory and cognitive performance.

During sleep, the brain has the ability to consolidate and process new information, helping to improve memory and learning. Additionally, sleep can help to reduce stress and anxiety, and improve overall mood.

4.**Supports physical health**: Adequate sleep is essential for physical health, as it helps to repair and restore the body. The body produces growth hormone while you're sleeping, which is essential for physical growth and development. Additionally, sleep can help to reduce inflammation and improve cardiovascular health.

5.**Promotes healthy weight**: Lack of sleep has been linked to obesity and weight gain, as it disrupts hormones that regulate appetite and metabolism. On the other hand, adequate sleep can help to regulate hormones and promote healthy weight.

To make sure you're sleeping as soundly as possible, consider the following tips:

1.**Stick to a routine**: Maintaining a consistent sleep schedule can help to regulate sleep patterns and improve the quality of sleep.

2. **Create a sleep-friendly environment**: Make sure that your bedroom is quiet, cool, and dark, and avoid using electronic devices before bedtime.

3. **Limit caffeine and alcohol consumption**: Caffeine and alcohol can interfere with sleep, so it's important to limit consumption, especially in the hours leading up to bedtime.

4. **Exercise regularly**: Regular physical activity can help to improve sleep quality and reduce stress and anxiety.

5. **Practice relaxation techniques**: Deep breathing, meditation, and yoga can all help to reduce stress and promote sleep.

Sleep is a crucial aspect of overall health and longevity, and ensuring that you are getting high-quality sleep is essential for maintaining physical and mental well-being. By making sleeping well a part of your daily routine, you can reduce the risk of developing sleep-related health problems and promote a longer, healthier life.

Here are a few additional points on the importance of sleep and its relationship to longevity:

1. **Chronic sleep deprivation can increase the risk of chronic diseases**: Chronic lack of sleep can lead to a range of health problems, including heart disease, diabetes, and stroke. The reason for this is that lack of sleep can throw off the hormone balance and chemicals in the body, leading to inflammation and oxidative stress, which may increase the risk of chronic diseases.

2. **Sleep affects mental health**: Poor sleep can impact mental health, leading to symptoms of anxiety, depression, and irritability. On the other hand, good sleep can help to reduce stress and improve overall mood, leading to better mental health and overall well-being.

3. **Sleep and aging**: As we age, our sleep patterns often change, leading to less sleep and less deep sleep. This can have a significant impact on overall health and longevity, as it can increase the risk of developing chronic diseases and impair brain function.

4. **The role of sleep in weight management**: Lack of sleep can disrupt hormones that regulate appetite and metabolism, leading to weight gain. On the other hand, good sleep can help to regulate hormones, improve metabolism, and promote healthy weight management.

5. **Importance of adequate sleep**: It's important to ensure that you are getting adequate sleep each night, and not just quality sleep. Adults should sleep for 7-9 hours each night, according to the National Sleep Foundation, while older adults may require slightly less.

In addition to these points, it's also worth noting that sleep quality and quantity can be affected by various factors, including sleep disorders, medical conditions, stress, and lifestyle habits. If you are struggling with sleep, it's important to talk to your doctor to rule out any underlying medical conditions and to get personalized advice on how to improve your sleep.

CHAPTER 5

Mindfulness and Longevity: Cultivating a Positive Mindset

The use of mindfulness has been shown to have a positive impact on overall health and well-being, including longevity. Here are some important things to think about when it comes to mindfulness and longevity:

1.**Mindfulness and stress reduction**: Mindfulness practices, such as meditation and deep breathing, have been shown to be effective in reducing stress and anxiety. This is because mindfulness helps to quiet the mind and promote a state of relaxation, which can help to reduce the physical and psychological effects of stress.

2.**Mindfulness and chronic disease**: Research has shown that mindfulness practices can have a positive impact on chronic diseases, such as heart disease, high blood pressure, and diabetes. This is because mindfulness can help to reduce inflammation and oxidative stress, which are major contributing factors to the development of these conditions.

3.**Mindfulness and brain health**: Mindfulness practices have been shown to improve brain function, including memory, attention, and executive function. This is likely because mindfulness helps to increase blood flow to the brain, which can improve cognitive function and reduce the risk of age-related brain decline.

4. **Mindfulness and positive emotions**: Mindfulness practices can help to increase positive emotions, such as happiness and contentment. This is because mindfulness helps to cultivate a positive mindset and reduce negative thoughts, leading to greater overall well-being.

5. **Incorporating mindfulness into daily life**: Mindfulness practices can be incorporated into daily life in a variety of ways, including through formal meditation practices, breathing exercises, and mindful activities, such as yoga or tai chi. It's important to find the type of mindfulness practice that works best for you and to make it a regular part of your routine.

In addition to these points, it's important to remember that mindfulness practices take time and effort to develop and that it's normal for the mind to wander during meditation. With practice, however, mindfulness can become a valuable tool in promoting overall health and longevity. If you want to incorporate mindfulness into your life, it may be helpful to work with a qualified mindfulness teacher or therapist who can help guide you through the process.

Here are more points to consider when it comes to mindfulness and longevity:

1. **The role of epigenetics**: Recent research has shown that mindfulness practices can affect epigenetics, which are the

molecular changes that occur in response to environmental factors. These changes can affect gene expression, leading to a variety of positive health outcomes, including increased longevity.

2.**The relationship between mindfulness and inflammation**: Inflammation is a key factor in many chronic diseases and is also associated with aging. Research has shown that mindfulness practices can help to reduce inflammation, which can in turn reduce the risk of chronic disease and promote longevity.

3.**Mindfulness and telomere length**: Telomeres are the protective caps at the end of our chromosomes that shorten as we age. Telomere length has been linked to a higher risk of age-related diseases and decreased lifespan. Research has shown that mindfulness practices can help to increase telomere length, which can promote longevity.

4.**Mindfulness and resilience**: Mindfulness practices can help to increase resilience, which is the ability to adapt to stress and bounce back from adversity. This is because mindfulness helps to increase positive emotions and reduce negative thoughts, allowing individuals to better handle stressful situations.

5. **Mindfulness and heart health**: Heart disease is a leading cause of death worldwide. According to research, mindfulness techniques can be beneficial on heart health, including reducing blood pressure and improving heart rate variability.

These are only a few examples in which mindfulness practices can promote longevity and overall health. By incorporating mindfulness into daily life and making it a regular part of your routine, you can reap the benefits of this powerful practice for years to come.

CHAPTER 6

Relationships and Longevity: Building Strong Connections

Relationships are essential to our lives, and research has shown that they can also impact our longevity. Strong relationships can provide social support, reduce stress, and promote overall well-being. Here are a few ways that relationships can promote longevity:

1.**Social support**: Studies have shown that people who have strong social support systems are more likely to live longer and experience better health outcomes. Relationships provide us with a sense of belonging, which can help us to feel connected and reduce feelings of loneliness and isolation.

2.**Reducing stress**: Strong relationships can help to reduce stress, which can have negative effects on our health. Social support can help to buffer the negative effects of stress by providing a sense of security and reducing feelings of worry and anxiety.

3.**Promoting healthy behaviors**: Relationships can also have a positive impact on our health behaviors. For example, having a supportive partner can encourage us to make healthier lifestyle choices, such as exercising regularly and eating a nutritious diet.

4. **Positive emotions**: Relationships can also increase positive emotions, such as happiness, which has been linked to better health outcomes and increased longevity.

5. **Reducing risk factors**: Research has shown that people with strong social support systems are less likely to engage in risky behaviors, such as smoking or excessive alcohol consumption.

It's important to note that not all relationships are equal in their impact on our health. Research has shown that the quality of our relationships is more important than the quantity. For example, a close relationship with a partner, family member, or close friend is likely to have a greater impact on our health than many weak or casual relationships.

Building strong relationships takes effort, but the rewards are worth it. By investing time and energy into our relationships, we can create strong connections that provide social support, reduce stress, and promote longevity.

In addition to the benefits outlined above, research has shown that relationships can also have a positive impact on our physical health. For example:

1. **Cardiovascular health**: Strong social support has been linked to better cardiovascular health. People who have

strong relationships are less likely to develop high blood pressure, heart disease, and other cardiovascular issues.

2.**Mental health**: Relationships can also improve our mental health. People who have a lot of social support are less likely to experience depression, anxiety, and other mental health issues.

3.**Immune system**: Relationships can also have a positive impact on our immune system. Research has shown that people with strong social support have stronger immune systems and are less likely to get sick.

4.**Cognitive function**: Strong relationships can also help to promote cognitive function and delay the onset of age-related conditions, such as dementia and Alzheimer's disease.

5.**Chronic conditions**: People with strong social support systems are also less likely to develop chronic conditions, such as obesity, diabetes, and other health issues.

Additionally, it's crucial to keep in mind that the standard of our relationships can have a positive or negative impact on our health. For example, a toxic relationship can increase stress, negative emotions, and increase the risk of developing health problems. On the other hand, strong, supportive relationships can provide us with the social support and positive emotions that promote longevity.

In conclusion, relationships play an important role in our health and well-being, and can impact our longevity. By investing time and energy into our relationships, we can create strong connections that provide social support, reduce stress, and promote overall well-being.

CHAPTER 6

Environmental Factors and Longevity: Living in Harmony with Nature

Environmental factors play a crucial role in our health and longevity. Research has shown that exposure to toxic substances and pollution, as well as living in an environment that lacks access to nature, can have negative impacts on our health. On the other hand, living in an environment that is supportive and in harmony with nature can promote overall health and well-being.

Here are some of the ways that environmental factors can impact our longevity:

1. **Exposure to toxic substances**: Exposure to toxic substances, such as air pollution, chemicals, and pesticides, can lead to a range of health problems, including respiratory problems, cardiovascular disease, and certain types of cancer.

2. **Access to nature**: Access to green spaces, such as parks and nature reserves, can have a positive impact on our health and well-being. Research has shown that spending time in nature can help to reduce stress, promote mental well-being, and boost our immune system.

3. **Living conditions**: Living conditions, such as overcrowding and poor housing, can also have a negative impact on our health. Overcrowding can lead to increased stress levels, while poor housing can result in exposure to toxic substances and other health hazards.

4. **Climate change**: Climate change is also having a major impact on our health and longevity. Rising temperatures, increased frequency of natural disasters, and changes in the distribution of disease-carrying insects can all have negative impacts on our health.

By taking steps to reduce exposure to toxic substances, spending time in nature, and living in an environment that supports health and well-being, we can improve our longevity and overall quality of life. This may include:

1. **Reducing exposure to toxins**: Taking steps to reduce exposure to toxic substances, such as using natural and non-toxic products, and choosing to live in an area with low levels of pollution.

2. **Spending time in nature**: Incorporating time spent in nature into your daily routine, such as going for a walk in the park, or taking a hike in the woods.

3. **Living in supportive environments**: Seeking out living conditions that promote health and well-being, such as living in a community with access to green spaces and healthy food options.

4. **Supporting environmental sustainability**: Supporting environmental sustainability through actions such as reducing energy consumption, using eco-friendly products, and supporting policies that promote a healthy environment.

Environmental factors play a crucial role in our health and longevity. By taking steps to live in an environment that is supportive and in harmony with nature, we can improve our overall well-being and increase our chances of living a long, healthy life.

Here are some additional ways that we can support our health and longevity through our environment:

1. **Active transportation**: Choosing active forms of transportation, such as walking or cycling, can help to reduce exposure to air pollution, while also providing an opportunity for physical activity.

2. **Indoor air quality**: Improving indoor air quality by using natural and non-toxic products, and ensuring proper ventilation can help to reduce exposure to toxic substances and improve overall health.

3. **Community design**: Supporting community design that promotes physical activity, such as providing access to green

spaces and safe walking and cycling paths, can encourage physical activity and promote overall health.

4.**Sustainable food systems**: Supporting sustainable food systems, such as local and organic agriculture, can help to reduce exposure to toxic substances, while also promoting healthy diets and supporting environmental sustainability.

5.**Green buildings**: Encouraging the use of green building practices, such as using energy-efficient materials, and promoting the use of natural light, can help to reduce exposure to toxins and improve indoor air quality.

By taking a holistic approach to our environment, we can support our health and longevity and help to create a more sustainable and healthier world for future generations. This may include supporting policies that promote sustainability, investing in green technologies, and advocating for environmentally-friendly practices in our communities.

In addition, it's important to keep in mind that our individual actions can have a significant impact on the environment. By making small changes in our daily lives, such as reducing energy consumption, choosing eco-friendly products, and supporting sustainable food systems, we can make a positive impact on the environment and our own health.

CHAPTER 7

Supplements and Longevity: Navigating the World of Anti-Aging

Supplements and longevity are often linked, as people seek ways to slow down the aging process and maintain their health and vitality. However, navigating the world of anti-aging supplements can be challenging, as there is a wide range of products available and limited regulation of their quality and efficacy.

It is important to remember that supplements should not be considered a replacement for a healthy diet and lifestyle. A balanced diet that includes plenty of fruits and vegetables, whole grains, and lean protein, along with regular physical activity and stress management, can provide all the nutrients and support that the body needs for optimal health and longevity.

However, for some individuals, taking certain supplements may help to support their health and well-being. Here are some commonly used anti-aging supplements and the potential benefits they may offer:

1. **Antioxidants**: Antioxidants such as vitamins C and E, beta-carotene, and selenium may help to protect the body from oxidative damage caused by free radicals, which can contribute to aging and disease.

2. **Omega-3 fatty acids**: Omega-3 fatty acids found in fish oil may help to support heart health, reduce inflammation, and protect against age-related diseases.

3. **Vitamin D**: Vitamin D is essential for bone health and may also play a role in maintaining overall health and reducing the risk of certain diseases.

4. **Resveratrol**: Resveratrol, a compound found in red wine, may help to reduce oxidative stress and improve heart health.

5. **Coenzyme Q10 (CoQ10)**: CoQ10 is a naturally-occurring enzyme that plays a role in energy production and may help to protect against cellular damage and support cardiovascular health.

It is crucial to consult a healthcare professional before starting any new supplement regimen, as some supplements can interact with medications or have other side effects. In addition, it is important to look for supplements that are third-party tested for quality and purity, as the supplement industry is largely unregulated and some products may not contain the active ingredients listed on their labels.

Ultimately, while supplements may offer some potential benefits for longevity, they should be seen as a complement to a healthy diet and lifestyle, rather than a replacement for these important habits. By focusing on overall health and well-being, we can help to support our longevity and live a long, healthy, and fulfilling life.

It is crucial to remember that the effects of anti-aging supplements can vary from person to person, and that not all supplements are suitable for everyone. Some individuals may be more susceptible to certain side effects or health risks, and certain supplements may not be appropriate for individuals with certain medical conditions or who are taking certain medications.

In addition to speaking with a healthcare professional, individuals can also look for scientific studies and clinical trials that have evaluated the safety and efficacy of specific supplements. While some studies may have shown promising results, it is important to remember that results from individual studies should be taken with a grain of caution and that more research is often needed before conclusions can be made.

When it comes to maintaining longevity, the best approach is a holistic one that takes into account the entire spectrum of health and well-being. This includes not only a balanced diet and regular exercise, but also stress management, quality sleep, and positive relationships with loved ones. By incorporating these habits into our daily routines, we can help to support our health and well-being, and reduce the risk of age-related diseases and health issues.

It is also worth considering the role that environmental factors play in our health and longevity. Exposure to toxins and pollutants in the environment can have a negative impact on our health and contribute to aging and disease. By taking steps to reduce our exposure to these harmful substances and living in harmony with nature, we can help to support our health and well-being, and maintain a strong and resilient body and mind.

The topic of supplements and longevity is a complex one, and individuals seeking to support their health and well-being through supplementation should approach this topic with caution and seek the guidance of a healthcare professional. By focusing on overall health and well-being, and incorporating a holistic approach to our daily habits and routines, we can help to support our longevity and live a long, healthy, and fulfilling life.

In conclusion, the journey towards longevity is a complex and multi-faceted one that involves taking care of our physical, mental, and emotional health. By embracing a holistic approach and incorporating habits such as a healthy diet, regular exercise, stress management, quality sleep, and positive relationships, we can help to support our health and well-being, and reduce the risk of age-related diseases and health issues.

It is also important to recognize the role that environmental factors play in our health and longevity, and to take steps to reduce our exposure to harmful toxins and pollutants. And, while the use of anti-aging supplements can be a tempting solution, it is important to approach this topic with caution and seek the guidance of a healthcare professional.

Ultimately, the key to embracing the journey to longevity is to focus on overall health and well-being, and to cultivate a positive mindset that emphasizes balance and harmony. By doing so, we can support our longevity and live a long, healthy, and fulfilling life.

In addition to these practical steps, it is also important to embrace a growth mindset and to continue learning and expanding our knowledge and understanding of health and wellness. By staying up-to-date with the latest research and trends, and by continually seeking out new and innovative solutions, we can help to support our health and longevity, and to live our lives to the fullest.

So, embrace the journey to longevity with confidence and optimism, and look forward to a future filled with health, happiness, and fulfillment. With a holistic approach and a commitment to overall health and well-being, the possibilities for a long and fulfilling life are endless.

www.ingramcontent.com/pod-product-compliance
Lightning Source LLC
Chambersburg PA
CBHW070318240526
45467CB00046B/1999